PEGAN DIET

*Why Is It Called The Pegan Diet
And What It Is*

kim louis

1

Table of Contents

Chapter 1

what is a pegan diet regimen?

The pegan concept is a nutrient-rich diet regimen that includes regarding 75% plant-based foods, with the staying 25% of your nourishment from pet resources. It tensions consuming entire, fresh foods that are sustainably generated, with restricted results on the atmosphere. The diet regimen additionally restrictions refined foods.

Why is it called the pegan diet regimen?

Pegan, both word and diet regimen, was developed in 2014 by

Dr. Note Hyman. It's a mix of paleo and vegan diet regimens, thus the call. Put simply, the pegan diet regimen enables lean meats, oily fish, and eggs (usually not allowed in veganism) in addition to some grains and beans (stayed clear of by paleo eaters).

What is the pegan diet?

The pegan diet regimen integrates crucial concepts from paleo as well as vegan diet plans based upon the idea that nutrient-dense, entire foods can minimize swelling, stabilize blood sugar level, as well as assistance ideal health and wellness.

If your initially idea is that going paleo as well as vegan concurrently appears virtually difficult, you are not the only one.

In spite of its call, the pegan diet regimen is one-of-a-kind as well as has its very own establish of standards. Actually, it is much less limiting compared to either a paleo or vegan diet regimen on its own.

Significant focus is positioned on veggies as well as fruit, yet consumption of tiny to modest quantities of meat, particular fish, nuts, seeds, as well as some legumes is likewise permitted.

Greatly refined sugars, oils, as well as grains are prevented — yet still appropriate in really tiny quantities.

The pegan diet regimen is not made as a common, temporary diet regimen. Rather, it goals to be more lasting so that one could comply with it forever.

summary

The pegan diet regimen, while based upon concepts from both paleo as well as vegan diet plans, complies with its very own rubric as well as is made to be lasting over the long-term.

Foods to consume

The pegan diet regimen focuses highly on entire foods, or foods that have actually gone through little bit to no refining previously they make it in your plate.

Consume great deals of plants

The key food team for the pegan diet regimen is veggies as well as fruit — these ought to consist of 75% of your complete consumption.

Low-glycemic vegetables and fruits, such as berries as well as non-starchy veggies, ought to be stressed in get to reduce your blood sugar level feedback.

Tiny quantities of starchy veggies as well as sweet fruits might be enabled those that have actualy currently attained healthy and balanced blood sugar level manage before beginning the diet regimen.

Pick sensibly sourced healthy protein

Although the pegan diet regimen mostly highlights grow foods, sufficient healthy protein consumption from pet resources is still urged.

Keep in mind that since 75% of the diet regimen is comprised of veggies as well as fruit, much less compared to 25% continues to be for animal-based healthy proteins. Thus, you will have actually a a lot reduce meat consumption compared to you would certainly on a common paleo diet regimen — yet still greater than on any kind of vegan diet regimen.

The pegan diet regimen discourages consuming conventionally farmed meats or eggs. Rather, it locations focus on grass-fed, pasture-raised resources of beef, pork, fowl, as well as entire eggs.

It likewise motivates consumption of fish — especially those that have the tendency to have actually reduced mercury articles like sardines as well as wild salmon.

Adhere to minimally refined fats

On this diet regimen, you ought to consume healthy and balanced fats from particular resources, such as:

Nuts: Other than peanuts

Seeds: Other than refined seed oils

Avocado as well as olives: Cold-pressed olive as well as avocado oil might likewise be utilized

Coconut: Raw coconut oil is allowed

Omega-3s: Particularly those from low-mercury fish or algae

Grass-fed, pasture-raised meats as well as entire eggs likewise add to the fat articles of the pegan diet regimen.

Some entire grains as well as legumes might be eaten

Although the majority of grains as well as legumes are prevented on the pegan diet regimen as a result of their possible to affect blood sugar level, some gluten-free entire grains as well as legumes are allowed in restricted amounts.

Grain consumption ought to not surpass greater than a 1/2 mug (125 grams) each dish, while legume consumption ought to not surpass 1 mug (75 grams) daily.

Right below are some grains as well as legumes that you could possibly consume:

Grains: Black rice, quinoa, amaranth, millet, teff, oats

Legumes: Lentils, chickpeas, black beans, pinto beans

Nonetheless, you ought to more limit these foods if you have actually diabetic issues or another problem that adds to bad blood sugar level manage.

summary

The pegan diet regimen is comprised of 75% vegetables and fruits. The staying 25% is split mostly amongst meats, eggs, as well as healthy and balanced fats, such as nuts as well as seeds. Some legumes as well as gluten-free entire grains might be allowed restricted amounts.

Foods to prevent

The pegan diet regimen is more versatile compared to a paleo or vegan diet regimen since it enables periodic consumption of nearly any kind of food.

That claimed, numerous foods as well as food teams are highly prevented. A few of these foods are recognized to be harmful, while others might be thought about really healthy and balanced — relying on which you ask.

These foods are generally prevented on the pegan diet regimen:

Milk: Cow's milk, yogurt, as well as cheese are highly prevented. Nonetheless, foods made from sheep or goat milk are allowed in restricted amounts. Often grass-fed butter is permitted, also.

Gluten: All gluten-containing grains are highly prevented.

Gluten-free grains: Also grains that do not include gluten are prevented. Tiny quantities of gluten-free entire grains might be allowed periodically.

Legumes: The majority of legumes are prevented as a result of their possible to boost blood sugar level. Low-starch legumes, such as lentils, might be allowed.

Sugar: Any kind of create of included sugar, improved or otherwise, is typically prevented. It might be utilized periodically — yet really moderately.

Improved oils: Improved or very refined oils, such as canola, soybean, sunflower, as well as corn oil, are often prevented.

Food ingredients: Fabricated colorings, flavorings, chemicals, as well as various other ingredients are prevented.

A lot of these foods are prohibited as a result of their regarded effect on blood sugar level as well as/or swelling in your body.

summary

The pegan diet regimen discourages numerous foods as well as food teams. Nonetheless, it's rather versatile. Restricted quantities of outlawed foods might be permitted periodically.

Possible drawbacks

Regardless of its favorable connects, the pegan diet plan likewise has some drawbacks that deserve taking into consideration.

Unneeded constraints

Although the pegan diet plan permits more versatility compared to a vegan or paleo diet plan alone, a number of the recommended constraints needlessly restrict really healthy and balanced foods, such as legumes, entire grains, as well as milk.

Supporters of the pegan diet plan frequently point out raised swelling as well as raised blood sugar level as the main factors for the elimination of these foods.

Certainly, many people do have hatreds gluten as well as milk that can advertise swelling. In a similar way, particular people have a hard time to manage blood sugar level when eating high-starch foods like grains or legumes.

In these instances, minimizing or getting rid of these foods could be ideal.

Nevertheless, unless you have particular allergic reactions or intolerances, it is unneeded to stay clear of them.

In addition, approximate removal of big teams of foods can result in vitamins and mineral shortages if those nutrients typically aren't very meticulously changed. Therefore, you could require a standard recognizing of nourishment to execute the pegan diet plan securely.

Absence of ease of access

Although a diet regimen filled with natural fruits, veggies, as well as grass-fed, pasture-raised meats could appear terrific theoretically, it could be unattainable for many individuals.

For the diet plan to be effective, you require considerable time to commit to dish preparation, some experience with food preparation as well as dish preparation, as well as accessibility to a range of foods that could be rather costly.

In addition, because of the constraints on usual refined foods, such as food preparation oils, eating in restaurants could be tough. This might possibly result in raised social seclusion or stress and anxiety.

Recap

The pegan diet plan needlessly limits a number of healthy and balanced food teams. It could likewise be costly as well as time eating.

Example food selection

The pegan diet plan stresses veggies however likewise consists of sustainably increased meats, fish, nuts, as well as seeds. Some legumes as well as gluten-free grains could be utilized moderately.

Scientists have examined vegan diet plans and also fat burning as well. Many just lately, a 2022 research released in the journal Excessive weight Scientific research and also Exercise, located that individuals that took place a low-fat, vegan diet regimen for 16 weeks did "reduce body weight, body make-up, and also insulin level of sensitivity."

Is fat burning feasible?

If you are seeking to lose some extra pounds, you could possibly have thought about attempting a vegan diet regimen. Vegans do not consume meat, fish, eggs, or milk items. Rather, they consume points like fresh vegetables and fruits, beans and also legumes, along with plant-based milks, various other nondairy items, and also meat choices.

Although lot of individuals pick the vegan way of life from ethical problems for pets, the diet regimen itself can have some health and wellness advantages. Inning accordance with current research researches, being vegan could also aid you shed a substantial quantity of weight.

How precisely? More research study is required, yet it is idea that going vegan could cause decreasing the variety of high-calorie foods you take in. With a vegan diet regimen, you could possibly wind up changing such foods with high-fiber choices that are reduced in calories and also maintain you fuller much longer.

Yet is this method healthy and balanced?

Reducing out a few of the primary food teams in your diet regimen could appear harmful. And also unless you very meticulously take note of your nourishment, it can be.

Some concern, for instance, concerning obtaining sufficient healthy protein or various other vital nutrients, like vitamin B-12. This vitamin is located normally just in pet items, and also if you ended up being deficient, it could lead to anemia. Vegans have to supplement their diet regimen with vitamins, vitamin-fortified cereals, and also strengthened soy items to prevent shortages.

Others could have difficulty with yo-yo weight loss after going vegan. What does this indicate? It is when you experience cycles of reducing weight and afterwards regaining all or more of that weight, potentially after having actually difficulty sticking to vegan-only foods. This kind of weight loss is related to some significant health and wellness effects, like an enhanced threat for kind 2 diabetes mellitus and also heart problem.

No matter these and also various other feasible challenges, you can consume a vegan diet regimen healthily and also drop weight. The essential — just like all diet plans — is concentrating on nutrient-dense foods versus vacant calories. For vegans, these foods would certainly consist of points like:

fresh vegetables and fruits

entire grains

beans and also legumes

nuts and also seeds

Restrict or prevent vegan refined foods which contain these included components:

fats

sugars

starches

salt

food ingredients

Pointers for fat burning

Ladies usually have to consume 2,000 calories every day to keep weight. To drop weight, this number decreases to about 1,500 calories a day. Guys usually have to consume 2,500 calories every day to keep their weight and also about 2,000 calories a day to drop weight.

A junk-food calorie does not equivalent a whole-food calorie regarding nourishment goes. Also if you remain listed below your calorie objective, filling out on all Nutter Butter cookies, which occur to be vegan, is extremely various from filling out on pails of fresh create.

There are lots of elements that impact fat burning, consisting of:

age

elevation

existing weight

diet regimen

exercise degrees

metabolic health and wellness

various other clinical problems

Although you can not regulate all these elements, you can regulate your diet regimen and also workout. No matter the kind of diet regimen you pick, you ought to comply with these standards for healthy and balanced consuming.

1. Time your dishes

Grazing throughout the day isn't really great for fat burning. Timing your dishes is important to increasing your metabolic process and also advertising healthy and balanced consuming routines.

Generally, attempt consuming dishes at the very same time every day to obtain your mind and also belly into a foreseeable pattern. Munch on a bigger morning meal in contrast to the various other dishes in your day. This could indicate changing your lunch a little bit previously and also consuming a smaller sized supper.

If you have exercised, attempt consuming within 45 mins of ending up. This will aid feed and also fixing your muscle mass.

When should not you consume? Within 2 hrs of going to bed. Eating calories as well near going to bed is related to weight acquire and also rest disruptions.

2. View your sections

Section dimensions issue with any one of the foods you consume — vegan or otherwise. The Joined Mentions Division of Agriculture's My Plate recommends that ordinary females and males obtain the adhering to variety of servings of these foods every day:

The very same policies put on vegan and also non-vegan treats: Consume them in small amounts. The ordinary American consumes a tremendous 22.2 teaspoons of sugar every day. Whether that originates from a decadent gelato sundae or a set of vegan cookies, it is still 335 calories which contain bit dietary worth.

Sugar can really interrupt your metabolic process and also cause health and wellness problems past weight acquire, consisting of hypertension, swelling, and also raised blood triglycerides. Just what does it cost? of the wonderful things suffices? Ladies ought to aim to restrict their day-to-day sugars to about 6 teaspoons or 100 calories every day. Guys ought to purpose to obtain less compared

to 9 teaspoons or 150 calories
every day.

If you are seeking a healthy and
balanced vegan treat

alternative

that is reasonably reduced in
calories without included sugars
and also fats, attempt fresh fruit.
Or else, consume a little section of
a vegan treat and also conserve the
remainder for tomorrow or
following week.

All-time low line

Consuming a vegan diet regimen could aid you drop weight. Still, it is constantly a smart idea to speak with your medical professional or a dietitian previously production huge modifications for a diet regimen. You ought to review how you will obtain important nutrients, like healthy protein and also B vitamins.

Your medical professional could likewise have various other recommendations for how you could drop weight, like maintaining a food diary or taking part in a routine workout regular.

3. See to it you are obtaining sufficient healthy protein

Present suggestions for healthy protein consumption are about 5.5 ounces daily, or about 0.41 grams each extra pound of body weight. This indicates a 150-pound female need to eat about 61 grams of healthy protein daily. A 175-pound male need to eat about 72 grams daily.

When you damage this down into calories, there have to do with 4 calories each gram of healthy protein. So the female in this instance would certainly should obtain 244 calories from healthy protein daily, and the male would certainly should obtain 288 calories from healthy protein.

4. Hand down "healthy and balanced" beverages

In the past you sip that store-bought smoothie, take into consideration the amount of calories it could consist of. Also supposed healthy and balanced beverages and power blends can load fairly a caloric strike.

Initially, let's have a look at a drink lots of people understand to guide remove while weight loss: A 20-ounce soft drink consists of about 240 calories and 15 to 18 teaspoons of sugar.

Yet what regarding that fresh pressed orange juice? It consists of regarding 279 calories each 20 ounces. That acai smoothie? It might consist of 460 calories each 20 ounces.

Review tags very meticulously and take into consideration conserving these beverages for unique celebrations.

Sticking with sprinkle is normally your best choice when attempting to decrease the number on the range. It is hydrating and consists of no calories. If you do not like simple sprinkle, you could take into consideration including a press of lemon or lime or attempting natural teas and shimmering waters.

5. Do not binge on plant-based treats.

The exact same policies relate to vegan and also non-vegan treats: Consume them in small amounts. The ordinary American consumes a tremendous 22.2 teaspoons of sugar daily. Whether that originates from a decadent gelato sundae or a set of vegan cookies, it is still 335 calories which contain little bit dietary worth.

Sugar can surely in fact interfere with your metabolic rate and also cause health and wellness concerns past weight acquire, consisting of hypertension, swelling, and also raised blood triglycerides. Just what does it cost? of the wonderful things suffices? Ladies must attempt to restrict their day-to-day sugars to about 6 teaspoons or 100 calories daily. Males must objective to obtain less compared to 9 teaspoons or 150 calories daily.

If you are searching for a healthy and balanced vegan treat

choice

that is fairly reduced in calories without included sugars and also fats, attempt fresh fruit. Or else, consume a tiny section of a vegan treat and also conserve the remainder for tomorrow or following week.

Chapter 2
Errors to Stay clear of on a Vegan or Vegan Diet regimen

A well balanced vegan or vegan diet regimen can possibly supply lots of health and wellness advantages.

These diet regimens have been connected with weight reduction, much far better blood glucose regulate, a lowered threat of heart problem and also a reduced threat of particular kinds of cancer cells.

Nevertheless, it can possibly be testing to keep a well-rounded vegan diet regimen that offers all the nutrients you require.

This write-up uncovers several of one of the most typical errors people make on a vegan or vegan diet regimen, and also the best ways to stay clear of them.

1. Thinking That Vegan or Vegan Items Are Immediately Much healthier

Regrettably, even if a foodstuff is classified "vegan" or "vegan" does not always suggest it is much healthier compared to the normal choice.

As an example, almond milk is a prominent, plant-based milk that is frequently a staple in vegan diet regimens.

Nevertheless, while almond milk is reduced in calories and also improved with numerous essential nutrients, it's not always much healthier compared to cow's milk.

As an example, 1 mug (240 ml) of low-fat cow's milk consists of 8 grams of healthy protein, while the exact same quantity of unsweetened almond milk consists of just 1 gram.

Sweetened almond milk can possibly additionally be high in included sugar, with 16 grams of sugar in simply 1 mug.

Various other vegan items, such as soy-based veggie burgers, nuggets and also meat options, are frequently very refined, with a lengthy listing of synthetic active ingredients. So they're frequently no much healthier compared to various other non-vegetarian refined foods.

In spite of being vegan, these items are additionally frequently high in calories, yet doing not have the healthy protein, fiber and also nutrients required for a well balanced dish.

While these items might reduce your shift to a vegan or vegan diet regimen, it is ideal to eat them in small amounts with a diet regimen abundant in nourishing, entire foods.

Recap: Lots of

foods marketed as vegan or vegan are frequently very refined, high in included

sugar or doing not have in nutrients. If you consist of these items in your diet regimen, consume

them just in small amounts.

2. Not Obtaining Sufficient Vitamin B12

Vitamin B12 plays numerous essential functions in the body. It is essential in the production of red blood cells and also DNA, to name a few procedures.

Regrettably, the major resources of vitamin B12 are pet items, such as meat, chicken, shellfish, eggs and also milk items.

Consequently, vegetarians have a raised threat of vitamin B12 shortage.

Vitamin B12 shortage can possibly create exhaustion, memory issues and also tingling. It can possibly additionally cause megaloblastic anemia, a problem brought on by having actually a lower-than-normal quantity of red blood cells.

Regrettably, a high consumption of folate can possibly really mask vitamin B12 shortage, concealing signs and symptoms up till the damages comes to be irreparable.

Nevertheless, there are foods and also supplements offered that can possibly assistance vegetarians fulfill their vitamin B12 requirements.

Besides pet items, strengthened foods and also particular kinds of edible algae additionally have vitamin B12.

Vegetarians must check their vitamin B12 consumption very meticulously and also take into consideration taking supplements if their requirements typically aren't fulfilled via diet regimen alone.

Recap: Vegetarians

and also vegans go to a higher threat of vitamin B12 shortage, so make certain you

eat strengthened foods or B12 supplements.

3. Changing Meat With Cheese

Among the most convenient methods to build almost any type of meal vegan is to obtain the meat and change it with cheese. When it involves taste, the switch functions well for sandwiches, salads, pasta and a lot of various other meals.

Nonetheless, while cheese does include a great quantity of healthy protein, minerals and vitamins, it does not change the broad variety of nutrients discovered in meat.

One ounce (28 grams) of beef, as an example, consists of 4 times the quantity of iron and dual the zinc discovered in one ounce of cheddar cheese.

Cheese additionally consists of much less healthy protein and more calories compared to meat.

As a matter of fact, ounce-for-ounce, cheese consists of just concerning 80% of the healthy protein discovered in hen, however almost 2.5 times the calories.

As opposed to just changing meat with cheese, you ought to consist of a selection of grow foods in your diet plan to satisfy your nutrition requirements.

Chickpeas, quinoa, tempeh, lentils, beans and nuts are all exceptional choices to provide help complete a vegan diet plan.

Recap: Rather

of simply changing meat with cheese, ensure to additionally consist of a varied vary

of grow foods in your diet plan to supply crucial nutrients.

4. Consuming As well Couple of Calories

A lot of foods and food teams are off-limits for vegans and

vegetarians, which can possibly make it testing for them to satisfy their calorie requirements.

As a matter of fact, vegans and vegetarians have the tendency to consume less calories compared to individuals that consume both meat and plants.

One examine contrasted the dietary top quality of 1,475 people's diet plans, consisting of vegans, vegetarians, vegetarians that consumed fish, individuals that consumed both meat and plants and individuals that consumed meat just as soon as a week.

Vegans had actually the most affordable calorie consumption throughout all the teams, taking in 600 less calories compared to individuals that consumed both meat and plants.

Vegetarians had actually a somewhat greater calorie consumption compared to vegans, however still eaten 263 less calories compared to individuals that consumed both meat and plants.

Calories are the major resource of power for the body, and your body requirements a particular total up to work. Limiting calories way too much can possibly result in a number of unfavorable negative effects, such as nutrition shortages, exhaustion and a slower metabolic process.

Recap: Vegans

and vegetarians have the tendency to have actually a reduced calorie consumption compared to individuals that consume meat and plants. If you are complying with either of these diet plans, ensure you are conference

your calorie requirements.

5. Not Consuming Sufficient Sprinkle

Consuming sufficient sprinkle is essential for everybody, however could be specifically crucial for those that consume a great deal of fiber, consisting of vegetarians and vegans.

Vegetarians have the tendency to have actually a greater fiber consumption, since fiber-rich legumes, veggies and entire grains are staples in a healthy and balanced vegan diet plan.

One examine discovered that individuals that consume both meat and plants consume concerning 27 grams of fiber daily, while vegans and vegetarians consume concerning 41 grams and 34 grams, specifically.

Consuming sprinkle with fiber is essential due to the fact that it can possibly assistance fiber relocate with the digestion system and avoid concerns like gas, bloating and irregularity.

Fiber usage is unbelievably crucial for wellness, and was connected to a reduced danger of heart problem, stroke, diabetic issues and excessive weight.

Present standards suggest females eat at the very least 25 grams of fiber daily, and guys eat at the very least 38 grams.

To ensure you are consuming sufficient sprinkle, consume when you really feel dehydrated, and spread out your sprinkle consumption throughout the day to remain moistened.

Recap: Vegans

and vegetarians generally consume a great deal of fiber. Consuming sufficient sprinkle can possibly assistance

avoid digestion troubles related to raised fiber consumption, such as gas,

bloating and irregularity.

Example food selection

The pegan diet plan highlights veggies yet additionally consists of sustainably elevated meats, fish, nuts, and seeds. Some legumes and gluten-free grains might be made use of moderately.

Here's an example food selection for one week on the diet plan:

Monday

Morning meal: Veggie omelet with
a basic green salad worn olive oil

Lunch: Kale salad with chickpeas,
strawberries, and avocado

Supper: Wild salmon patties with
roasted carrots, steamed broccoli,
and lemon vinaigrette

Tuesday

Morning meal: Pleasant potato "salute" covered with sliced avocado, pumpkin seeds, and lemon vinaigrette

Lunch: Bento box with steamed eggs, sliced turkey, raw veggie sticks, fermented pickles, and blackberries

Supper: Veggie stir-fry with cashews, onions, bell pepper, tomato, and black beans

Wednesday

Morning meal: Green smoothie with apple, kale, almond butter, and hemp seeds

Lunch: Remaining veggie stir-fry

Supper: Smoked shrimp and veggie kabobs with black rice pilaf

Thursday

Morning meal: Coconut and chia seed dessert with walnuts and fresh blueberries

Lunch: Combined green salad with avocado, cucumber, smoked poultry, and cider vinaigrette

Supper: Roasted beet salad with pumpkin seeds, Brussels sprouts, and sliced almonds

Friday

Morning meal: Deep-fried eggs, kimchi, and braised environment-friendlies

Lunch: Lentil and veggie stew with a side of sliced cantaloupe

Supper: Salad with radishes, jicama, guacamole, and grass-fed beef strips

Saturday

Morning meal: Over night oats with cashew milk, chia seeds, walnuts, and berries

Lunch: Remaining lentil-veggie stew

Supper: Roast pork loin with steamed veggies, environment-friendlies, and quinoa

Sunday

Morning meal: Veggie omelet with a basic green salad

Lunch: Thai-style salad rolls with cashew lotion sauce and orange pieces

Supper: Remaining pork loin and veggies

Recap

The pegan diet plan highlights a vegetable-heavy diet plan that additionally consists of healthy protein, healthy and balanced fats, and some fruit. Grains and legumes are consisted of, yet much less regularly.

All-time low line

The pegan diet plan is based upon paleo and vegan concepts — however it motivates some meat usage.

It highlights entire foods, particularly veggies, while mainly prohibiting gluten, milk, many grains, and legumes.

It is abundant in several nutrients that can possibly advertise ideal wellness yet might be also limiting for lots of people.

You can possibly provide this diet plan a aim to see exactly how your body reacts. If you are currently paleo or vegan and want customizing your diet plan, the pegan diet plan might be simpler to adapt to.